# 150 HACKS AND TIPS FOR EXPECTING MOTHERS

## ADVICE, HACKS, TRICKS & TIPS FOR EXPERIENCING PREGNANCY THE RIGHT WAY

### TARYN ACCARDO

**Disclaimer**

THE INFORMATION CONTAINED IN THIS BOOK IS BASED ON RESEARCH, TESTIMONY AND PERSONAL EXPERIENCE, UNLESS OTHERWISE STATED. IT SHOULD NOT BE USED AS A SUBSTITUTE FOR QUALIFIED MEDICAL ADVICE. HEALTH RELATED INFORMATION PROVIDED IN THIS BOOK IS FOR EDUCATIONAL AND ENTERTAINMENT PURPOSES ONLY. ALWAYS SEEK THE COUNCIL OF A QUALIFIED MEDICAL PRACTITIONER, FOR AN INDIVIDUAL CONSULTATION, BEFORE MAKING ANY SIGNIFICANT CHANGES TO YOUR DIET AND LIFESTYLE. THE AUTHOR AND PUBLISHER DISCLAIM RESPONSIBILITY FOR ANY ADVERSE EFFECTS THAT MAY RESULT FROM THE USE OR APPLICATION OF THE RECIPES AND INFORMATION WITHIN THIS BOOK. THE PUBLISHER AND AUTHOR MAKE NO REPRESENTATIONS OR WARRANTIES WITH RESPECT TO THE ACCURACY OR COMPLETENESS OF THE CONTENTS OF THIS WORK AND SPECIFICALLY DISCLAIM ALL WARRANTIES INCLUDING, WITHOUT LIMITATION, WARRANTIES OF FITNESS, HEALTH OR WEIGHT LOSS FOR A PARTICULAR PURPOSE. THIS WORK IS SOLD WITH THE UNDERSTANDING THAT THE PUBLISHER AND AUTHOR ARE NOT ENGAGED IN RENDERING MEDICAL OR OTHER PROFESSIONAL ADVICE AND NEITHER IS LIABLE FOR DAMAGES ARISING FROM IT.

# TABLE OF CONTENTS

# INTRODUCTION

## WHY I WROTE THIS BOOK?

Learning that you have created a baby is one of the most exciting and terrifying experiences that a human can go through. In approximately 38 weeks, you are going to be completely responsible for an infant and then a toddler and then a child and then a teenager – and even after that, the care, worry and love that you have for your adult procreation is a unique experience, understood only by parents.

Before you get there, however, there are still 38 weeks to endure where your body will change considerably to allow for the growth of the fetus in your womb. You will experience cravings for the first time, stretch-marks, back pain, morning sickness and overwhelming joy when your baby kicks or you see him or her growing in front of your eyes at each doctor's appointment.

The changes that your body experiences can sometimes be confusing or overwhelming and sometimes even a little scary. It's okay though, this book is here to ensure that you are physically, emotionally and mentally prepared. It has been written to help you feel as though you have a friend, right next to you, as you experience this brand new journey. It has been written as a guide and an assistant so you feel organized and ready for the big day.

We hope that it will serve as a comforting tool and informative resource that will assist you in making the most of a happy and healthy pregnancy.

## WHO IS THIS BOOK FOR?

This book is not simply for expecting mothers, but a resource for all of those who are involved in ensuring that when the baby is born, he or she is welcomed into the world by a happy, loving family and support network. You can be a pregnant mother, a partner, a parent to those expecting, a friend or even an individual who wants to reflect on your own experience as an expecting parent.

The advice in this book is incredibly beneficial but not limited to all of the above and is encouraged as a resource for anyone looking for more information on the hacks, tips, tricks and advice for a smooth and memorable pregnancy.

No matter who you are, you don't have to feel isolated at any stage of the journey that you are embarking on. You can also feel as if you and your support network are equipped with the information that will get you through the next few months, delivering you to D-day ready to embrace a new addition to the family. This is exciting time ahead and this book is here to steer you through it so that every corner, unexpected turn, speed bump, dead end and detour is anticipated and you're ready to handle it.

So buckle up, you're about to have the time of your life.

# CHAPTER 1 – BREAKING THE NEWS

## TO HIM

**001** You need to be calm when you break the news so take a bit of time to process it yourself. Are you excited or nervous? Was it planned or is it a surprise? Come to terms with what lies ahead and how you feel about it so that you can share the news from a clear place.

**002** What is his role in the future? Are you expecting him to be completely involved as a father raising a child, would you like financial support or are you looking for emotional support? Once you have evaluated your expectations, it will be easier to communicate these to him.

**003** Share the news slowly and in segments that are easy to digest. Try not to overwhelm him with all of your own emotions and expectations, allowing him time to come to terms with the news himself. Just like you, he may need a few moments to understand his own feelings and expectations.

**004** There is a possibility that he will react in shock or fear, which may not be the reaction that you expect or want. Try not to take it too personally if this happens. Give him some time to process the news.

**005** Have some fun. If the two of you have been trying to have a baby or you know that he'll love being a father, enjoy sharing the special news with him. Get him a shirt that says: 'I love daddy' or leave the pregnancy test somewhere that he will find it. The look on his face will be priceless.

## To Family

Some expecting mothers prefer to wait until their 8-week scan until the news spreads too far. Before the 8-week mark, the pregnancy is in a vulnerable stage and some people would prefer to wait until it is in a more stable stage before everyone knows about it. This is because if there are complications or a miscarriage, the trauma of telling everyone is lessened.

**006** It's natural to want to share this exhilarating news with your nearest and dearest. The greatest advantage to this is that you won't have to hide morning sickness, the fact that you are avoiding certain foods and alcohol or that you're expecting your life to change very soon.

**007** Telling your family early on will also mean that you have the necessary support that you need from day one. This could mean having someone to go to doctor's appointments with you, helping you to shop for baby or even just to massage your feet when your partner isn't around.

**008** Sharing the news with your family, just like sharing it with him, can be a creative and heart-warming experience. Bake a cake for a family function that says: 'We're expecting' or hand out little baby booties. You could even include a sonogram in a book that you pass around. Enjoy it, this is news that you will never forget sharing.

**009** Having a support network if there are complications or a miscarriage is important, however, so make sure to lean on the family who will offer you this. Family members who have experience with pregnancies and their own children can also offer advice and support from a place of knowing and understanding.

## To Friends

**010** When you're ready to share the news with your friends, whether it's before or after the 8-week mark, they can prove invaluable in their love, care and support. They'll also stop asking why you're holding back on the wine.

**011** Going completely public with the news that you're expecting is a delightful and thrilling process. There are also so many fun ways to do it, especially in the age of social media.

**012** Photographs can be great tools to share on Facebook or Twitter, which break the news. Share a photograph of your shoes, his shoes and a pair of baby booties in the middle. Share a photograph of him in a t-shirt that says, "I'm becoming a daddy on 02/05/2016". Or share a photograph of yourself reading a pregnancy magazine.

**013** Receiving your sonogram and watching your little one grow and develop in your womb is an exhilarating experience and one that is simple and effective to share with your friends. Post your scan on your favorite social media platform or email it to your best buddies. Figuring out where the head is will also be an entertaining experience for them.

**014** You could also just opt for the simple but effective method of announcing it in person to your friends. They will appreciate being told one-on-one and that the news is coming to them directly.

**015** Some of your friends may be trying and struggling to have a baby themselves. When you share the news with these friends, try to be sensitive to what they are going through at the time. While they will be overjoyed for you, it may be painful for them because they are desperate for their own baby. Give them some time and space to come to terms with your news.

# Chapter 2 – Build Your Network

## Professionals

**016** The most important professional in your life from the time that you find out that you are pregnant is your doctor. You may already have a regular doctor and if you suspect that you are pregnant, you should book an appointment with him or her immediately. Your doctor will test your blood, conduct routine pregnancy and health tests, discuss options with you and help you to choose where you want to have the baby.

**017** If you don't have a current doctor, there are a few ways to find one who you will feel comfortable with. Consult your support network of friends, family and colleagues as they may have a few recommendations for good doctors. You may also decide that you feel more comfortable with a male or female doctor. Consulting websites and directories of doctors in the area will also help you to locate one near to you. Book an appointment for as soon as possible.

**018** If your doctor is a General Practitioner, you may be referred to an Obstetrician or Gynecologist, who will be more specialized when it comes to healthcare for pregnancy. If you feel more comfortable with this, ask your GP to refer you to one or do some research on who the best are in your area. In America, there is a platform called The American Congress of Obstetricians and Gynecologists, which actually points doctors out on a map for you and provides up to date information and resources in women's health.

**019** You may also decide that you want a midwife to look after you during pregnancy and assist you with the birth of your baby. You can choose a certified nurse-midwife, who are trained in both nursing and midwifery, or a direct-entry midwife who is certified in midwifery and can assist with home births. Midwives are easy to find through referrals, word of mouth and birthing centers.

**020** Who you choose as your health care professional is entirely up to you and what you feel comfortable with, but get a few second opinions on the matter. If you have any health issues or risks, it may be better to use an Obstetrician or Gynecologist. Ensure that you have spoken thoroughly to your health care professional and know what all of the risks and advantages concerned. Do research on the matter, grow your network as much as possible so that you have all of the facts in front of you and decide on what you feel more comfortable with.

**021** Depression and anxiety are symptoms that many pregnant women experience and is something you do need to address with a professional. If you are feeling unnaturally down or anxious, don't simply write it off as the hormones. Tell your health care practitioner immediately how you are feeling. They will help you with therapy or even medication to make you feel better so that your pregnancy can be enjoyable as possible.

**022** When your baby is born, you will want a qualified pediatrician on hand to deliver the best pediatric health care to your precious child. Your healthcare practitioner will be able to recommend one that you and your baby will feel comfortable with.

## PERSONAL

**022** Your personal network is very important over the next nine months and even after that, when you welcome your infant into the world. You want to have like-minded people around you to support you and offer advice, love and care. Your friends and family can be your first port of call, but there are many other ways to grow your personal network.

**023** Antenatal classes are a fantastic way for you and your partner to prepare for the birth of your baby, while meeting people who are in a similar situation. Not only will you learn about labor, birth and being a parent but you will be sharing it with your partner and other parents. This provides a wonderful network with those who understand your excitement, worry and expectations.

**024** Word of mouth is a great way to build up a personal network of expecting parents and parents who understand what you are experiencing. Lean on your friends and family and ask them to introduce you to other pregnant couples. Spending time with families with small children will also help to prepare you for the little things that you don't even think of before you're a parent yourself.

**025** There might be a mom's walking group, a yoga class or a due-date club in your neighborhood so keep your eyes open for opportunities to bond. Combining exercise with meeting new people is a healthy way to stay active during pregnancy while expanding your personal networks.

**026** You may start to feel a little alienated or different to your friends who are not pregnant or don't have children yet. This is perfectly normal and often stems from a fear of relationships changing now that there is a baby bump in the mix. Communicate with your friends about how you are feeling and that you would still like to spend time with them, even if it's not at the pub. With some mutual respect and understanding, you'll be able to find common ground with them throughout your pregnancy.

## VIRTUAL

**027** In the age of social media and the internet, it is incredibly easy to build an online network to support you through your pregnancy. There are tons of online resources, groups and forums to assist you in your journey to motherhood. If you have access to the internet then it's as easy as 1, 2, 3.

**028** Facebook is a fantastic tool for meeting pregnant couples and parental support groups in your area, country or even the world. Type 'mom's group' or 'pregnant mom' into the search bar and you will see hundreds of options appear. Most of them are closed groups, but simply find the group you want to join and request to join it. Discussions around everything from morning sickness to doctor's visits are just a mouse click and an 'enter' key away.

**029** Online forums are another great way to interact with expecting moms and there are thousands out there. Try thebump.com, babyandbump.momtastic.com, netmums.com, justmommies.com, pregnancyforum.co.uk or simply type 'pregnancy forums' and the name of your country into the search bar. A virtual group of friends will be ready and waiting.

**030** If you're feeling sick, worried about a cramp or need some comforting advice, there is myriad of apps available for download on your phone that you can consult at any time during your pregnancy. The Babycenter app, for example, includes a community of other moms in the Birth Club as well as a nutrition guide. The growth widget will also show you how your baby is growing inside of you, making it easier to picture and imagine.

**031** There are also websites and apps dedicated to supporting pregnant mothers, including embraceherhealth.com, a "digital health education and support for women and moms". This is a rich health education tool, created by doctors. It also features online support from medical staff, taking patient engagement to a new level.

**032** The internet includes thousands of publications in the form of blogs, eBooks, websites, downloadable books and information packs to assist you with your pregnancy as well as parenthood. Read about people's real-life experiences dealing with pregnancy and parenthood, follow the blogs of those who are going through the exact same thing that you are going through right now and immerse yourself in the information and advice that they have to offer. Twitter is a great resource when it comes to keeping track of these authors, websites and books.

**033** YouTube is an incredibly useful virtual tool for tutorials, tips and advice when it comes to being a pregnant mom. You can build an entire network of your favorite moms sharing their experiences from day to day. You also won't feel alone as your body experiences changes, with a community of women sharing their stories right there with you.

# CHAPTER 3 – STAYING FIT

## KEEP MOVING

**034** On average a pregnant woman gains between 25 and 35 pounds over the nine months, so you want to remain as healthy and as fit as possible during your pregnancy. This not only makes it easier to shed the weight once baby is born but keeps you energetic, helps you to feel more comfortable, gets you ready for the birthing process, reduces your stress and will help you to sleep better.

**035** Staying fit during pregnancy can be as easy as going for a walk at least three times a week. Your pace will have to be fairly quick, but it's a gentle exercise that will get your heart pumping in a healthy way. The intensity and length of your walks depend on how fit you are and what trimester you are in but 30 minute walks are a good, average time.

**036** If running has been your exercise of choice, you can still partake when you are pregnant. It is good, however, to consult your doctor first about the intensity and length of your runs as it depends on the trimester that you are in. Running can put pressure on your knees so it's important to run within moderation and ensure that you aren't pushing yourself or training too hard.

**037** Swimming is a gentle way to stay fit, relieve any stress or pressure that your body is under and keep cool at the same time. Join an aerobics class or do laps in the pool using a pool noodle or floating device. This is a low impact exercise that is very good for your heart.

**038** Yoga is a wonderful way to remain supple and strong during pregnancy and you may even meet a few other moms-to-be while you're there. Many gyms and studios offer yoga classes designed for pregnant moms, so do some research in your area. Yoga keeps your flexible and improves your muscle tone.

**039** Dance classes or even putting some music on and showing off your moves in your own living room can get your heart pumping while toning your muscles at the same time. Check what classes your local gym offers, especially for expecting mothers, or pump up the tunes in your home. Be careful not to do any dance moves that are too strenuous on your body however, such as kicks or jumps.

**040** Aerobics is very good for your heart as well the muscles in your body, but you need to aim for low-impact classes designed for pregnant mothers. With varying moves and fun music, it won't even feel like a workout.

**041** If you've always trained with weights then it is okay to continue, as long as you have consulted your doctor and reduced the amount of weight that you are lifting. Weight training will keep you strong and feeling good about your body image.

**042** Keep stretching throughout your pregnancy to alleviate those aches and pains. You'll be working your heart muscles and keeping your body flexible as it goes through all of the changes over the next nine months.

**043** While it is important to stay fit and healthy during your pregnancy, listen to your body. If you are feeling too tired or are pushing yourself too much, have a rest. You don't want to put any added strain on you or the baby. If you feel dizzy, experience chest pains, are having trouble breathing or feel short of breath, these could be signs that you need to stop exercising. Ensure that you are keeping your healthcare professional updated on the exercises that you are doing.

# CHAPTER 4 – DIET

## FOODS TO AVOID

**044** During the course of your pregnancy and while you are breastfeeding, there are certain foods that you need to avoid to ensure your safety and the safety of your baby.

**045** Meat or poultry that is raw or hasn't been cooked properly and cold meats that are kept in the fridge should be avoided. Uncooked meat may contain a parasite that causes a toxoplasmosis infection, which could damage your baby.

**046** Patés are also to be avoided during pregnancy, as well as liver of any kind. Liver can contain high quantities of Vitamin A, which in excess can be harmful to your baby.

**047** While fish is a good addition to a healthy diet, try to avoid fish such as marlin, shark or swordfish. You should also limit the amount of tuna that you eat due to the amount of mercury it contains. In general you should only eat two portions of fish that are high in oil in a week. Opt for cooked shellfish rather than raw shellfish.

048 Avoid soft cheeses that are made from unpasteurized milk such as blue cheeses, feta, Camembert and Brie.

**049** Avoid consuming more than 200mg of caffeine while you are pregnant as well as tobacco and alcohol.

**050** Speak to your health care practitioner about the vitamins that you should be taking as some vitamins in excess are not good for the baby.

## BREAKFAST

**051** You really are eating for two when you're pregnant, so you need to increase your daily intake of nutritional and nourishing foods to around 1200 kilojoules a day. Breakfast is the best way to get some health-packed food into your system.

**052** Fresh fruit is delicious, light and filled with fiber and vitamins so pack it into your breakfast for energy. It will also keep your digestive system regular. Eat a bowl of your favorite fresh fruit plain, make a smoothie or use it to top off cereal, oatmeal or yoghurt.

**053** Dairy contains calcium, which is the important for the development of healthy bones, teeth and muscles. While your baby is growing inside of you, feed your body with fresh, low-fat yoghurts and milks.

**054** Full up on whole grains such as oatmeal, whole-grain breakfast cereals or whole-wheat toast. Whole grains keeps you full because your body digests it much slower than sugary, refined foods. It also contains essential irons and nutrients that are important for you and baby during pregnancy.

**055** Protein is very important for the growth of your baby and a delicious addition to breakfast time. You can also get creative. Make different types of eggs each morning, from omelets to poached eggs to fried eggs to keep breakfast exciting. However, try to eat thoroughly cooked eggs to avoid the risk of salmonella. You can also get your protein from peanut butter or cottage cheese.

**056** If you're struggling to get breakfast down due to morning sickness or nausea, go for simple foods such as dry toast or boiled eggs. Try to eat what you can but if you can't manage, make up for it over the course of the day with balanced, wholesome meals. Also drink ginger tea to alleviate the nausea.

## LUNCH

**057** Balanced meals are the way to go for pregnancy so opt for those that include a variety of different foods so that you get all of the nutrients, vitamins and minerals that you and your baby need.

**058** You should eat at least five servings of fruit and vegetables each day so ensure your lunches are packed with these. Try tasty salads or vegetable soups or roast some hearty vegetables. You can also make fruity smoothies or vegetable juices to ensure you're consuming as much flavor and goodness as possible.

**059** Starches such as bread, potatoes, rice, pasta and noodles are an important to add to your lunches, as well as your other meals, for energy, vitamins and fiber. Similarly to breakfasts opt for whole grain starches. You can make delicious noodle dishes, pastas or sandwiches for a balanced meal.

**060** Add some cheese, as long as it is made from pasteurized milk, to your lunch meals for added calcium.

**061** Include a bit of protein in your meal each lunch time, whether it be eggs, chicken, fish, meat, beans, nuts or pulses. Make a boiled egg or chicken salad, or order a meat sandwich from your favorite lunch spot. Protein will keep your baby strong as he or she grows.

**062** When those cravings hit during the day or late at night, try to avoid food that is high in sugar and fats. Sugary foods will spike your blood sugar and cause you to put on unnecessary weight during your pregnancy. These include cream, crisps, cake, fizzy drinks, biscuits, chocolate, ice cream and pastries.

## DINNER

**063** On your dinner plate, you want to include a lot of fruit and vegetables, a lot of whole-grain starches, some dairy foods and some protein. Foods high in fat and sugar must be limited. A balanced dinner is the best type of dinner.

**064** Get creative with your dinners. Research some healthy and wholesome recipes for pregnancy online or within your network. The forums that you have joined will share tasty dinner ideas, tips and recipes while your personal networks may even be able to help you to make them.

**065** Invest in a pregnancy recipe book for new and exciting ideas, that include all of the foods and flavors that you are allowed to eat while you are pregnant.

**066** If you're going to be working or busy through some or most of your pregnancy opt for dinners that are easy and quick to make. You'll probably be tired and your body may be aching when you get home from work, but you don't want this to deter you from eating a nutritional and healthy supper. Cook big portions, freeze them and heat them up for supper or throw together something that takes minimal preparation time.

**067** If you're struggling with constipation during pregnancy, include more whole grains in your meals, especially at dinner. The fibre will help to keep you regular.

**068** From morning through to night, it is important to drink as much fluid as possible, including water and herbal teas. Keep a water bottle with you at all times and drink water or herbal teas with or after your dinner to stay hydrated.

**069** As your pregnancy progresses, you may experience heartburn and indigestion. To alleviate this, try to eat smaller meals throughout the day and a smaller meal at dinner-time. Don't eat dinner too close to bedtime either, as lying down soon after eating may cause discomfort.

## SNACKS

**070** Its okay to snack between meals but avoid reaching for the sugary and high fat treats.

**071** Snack on fruits between meals. They are ready-to-eat, will satisfy any sugar cravings and provide you with the nutrients and vitamins that you need.

**072** Treat yourself to some baked beans or peanut butter on whole wheat toast. It will provide you with the protein and the whole grains that your body is looking for.

**073** Carrots, celery and cucumber are delicious and crunchy as well as filling. Dip them in some humus or cottage cheese for added flavor.

**074** Sandwiches packed with salad and/or tuna or salmon are a healthy and filling snack.

**075** Low fat and low sugar yoghurts are delicious and provide you with the calcium that you and your baby need during pregnancy.

**076** Snack on hearty vegetable soups to fill your belly.

# Chapter 5 – Comfort

## Sleep & Rest

**077** Your body is working very hard during pregnancy to care for you and baby, which means you may feel more tired than normal. However, you may struggle to get the sleep and rest that you need. You may experience discomfort while you're lying down as the baby grows larger inside of your womb as well as the urge to go to the toilet more often than normal, due to the pressure on your bladder. Some women also experience shortness of breath, heartburn, constipation and aches, pains and cramps, disrupting their sleeping pattern. Stress and anxiety may also keep you awake.

**078** If you have trouble sleeping, do not resort to sleeping pills even if they are herbal. They are not safe for the baby. Talk to your healthcare professional for more details.

**079** Develop a routine sleeping pattern so that your body learns to 'shut down' at a certain time every day.

**080** Caffeine should be limited in general during pregnancy but avoid consuming it before bed. Opt for herbal teas or water instead but limit your intake of these too so that your bladder doesn't get too full just before you go to sleep.

**081** Find a comfortable position to sleep in, using pillows to support you if necessary. Sleeping on your left side is recommended as it alleviates pressure on your organs. Try not to sleep on your back.

**082** Learn how to relax, especially before bedtime. Take a warm bath, meditate or read a soothing book. Yoga is also a good way to handle stress during pregnancy as well as relax your body.

**083** Use a hot water bottle when you're cramping to soothe your body. Walk around for a bit to relieve cramps in your legs.

**084** Talk to your loved ones if you're feeling stressed or anxious. Your support network is there so that you do not feel alone. There is no need for sleepless nights spent worrying. If you are anxious about the birth, do some more reading or attend antenatal classes so that you feel prepared and ready.

**085** Naps during the day will help you to feel rested and relaxed so that you don't feel overtired or worn out during your pregnancy.

**086** Be gentle on yourself and listen to your body. When you're feeling tired or you experience cramps, rest and look after yourself.

## GETTING AROUND

**087** It is safe to travel locally and abroad while you are pregnant, but you might experience morning sickness in your first trimester or, in your third trimester, you may be very tired. Rest stops will help with this, whether you're travelling by car, bus or train. Try to limit the length of time that you spend travelling.

**088** Stay safe while you're travelling by using your seat belt or remaining seated while on a bus or in a train. Make sure the airbags are turned on in your car.

**089** Pregnant women are usually allowed to fly, except for their ninth month. It is important to check with your healthcare professional, however, before you do fly. You may get special permission to fly in your ninth month. The turbulence and narrow aisles may not be comfortable so try to choose an aisle seat if you can and fasten your seat belt at all times.

**090** You can travel by sea while you are pregnant, but the motion of the sea may cause you to feel nauseous. Check with your healthcare practitioner what medicines you can take for seasickness that are safe for pregnant women. It's also important to check that there is a medical professional on board, to assist you if need be.

**091** The most important thing is to be comfortable, whether you're travelling to work and back each day or are going on a longer trip. Wear comfortable shoes and loose clothing.

**092** If you're going on a longer trip, make sure you have a few nutritional snacks and liquids packed to keep you hydrated and nourished.

# Chapter 6 – Temporary or Lasting Effects

## Physical

**093** Your body will go through many changes during pregnancy so it's important to be prepared for both the temporary and lasting physical effects.

**094** During pregnancy, you will notice that your breast size will increase. The hormones pumping through your body are the reason for this, as they prepare your body for breastfeeding. You may even find, during the third trimester and when baby is born, that your breasts leak a yellow fluid called colostrum. Your breasts should return to normal size when you finish breastfeeding, but in the interim wear a very supportive maternity bra and use breast pads to avoid leaks. If your breasts are very swollen and tender, consult your healthcare professional.

**095** Stretch marks are an inevitable part of pregnancy as the skin around your stomach, buttocks, breasts and upper legs stretch to make room for your growing baby. Sometimes the skin will scar as it stretches. Rub bio-oil into the skin every day during pregnancy and after birth to avoid lasting scarring. Bio-oil can be found at your local pharmacy.

**096** You may notice other changes in your skin during pregnancy, such as darker nipples and facial pigmentation, called Chloasma or melisma Gravidarum. Some women also experience a dark line that runs from their belly button to their pubic bone, called the linea nigra. If you suffering from this, try to stay out of the sun or wear high SPF sun protection at all times. Also be sure to use cleansers and facial treatments that aren't too harsh on the skin. The pigmentation should fade after birth, once your hormones have regulated but consult a dermatologist if it does not.

**097** Your face, ankles or hands may become very swollen, especially as you approach the birth of your baby. This is perfectly normal and can be relieved by drinking plenty of fluid, avoiding caffeine as well as rest. When you're lying down, ensure that your feet are elevated on a pillow.

**098** Varicose veins may also rear their head during pregnancy, causing your veins to look dark in color as well as swollen. You'd commonly notice them in your legs and they occur due to the amount of blood being pumped through your body as well as your growing uterus. Avoid wearing tight trousers that restrict the blood flow in your legs. Exercising regularly and lying with your legs up against a wall may also improve circulation. They should return to normal after you give birth.

**099** Haemorrhoids are unfortunately another side effect of pregnancy and are the varicose veins in your buttocks. If you are struggling with constipation, the haemorrhoids may be aggravated. Use haemorrhoid cream to treat them and eat foods high in fibre to avoid constipation. If they persist after childbirth, consult your doctor as you may need surgical treatment.

**100** Pregnant women often suffer with a weak bladder during pregnancy due to pressure on the bladder as well as the pelvis. Some women experience urinary leaking when they sneeze or laugh too hard. Kegel exercises will help to strengthen the muscles in the pelvis. Go to the bathroom often to relieve your bladder and try to be close to one at all times.

## MENTAL

**101** Mood swings are normal part of pregnancy, due to the hormone changes in your body. You may find yourself laughing one moment and crying the next. Doctors recommend taking Vitamin B as well as getting plenty of exercise and rest. Try relaxation techniques throughout your pregnancy such as meditation or yoga.

**102** Depression and anxiety during pregnancy as well as post-natal depression may occur and should be treated by a qualified professional. Don't try to treat yourself if you are feeling extremely overwhelmed, depressed or anxious at any stage during pregnancy or after your baby is born, speak to your doctor immediately. Ensure that you lean on your support network and get a lot of rest.

**103** Insomnia is experienced by many pregnant women and is the result of many things including discomfort, worrying about the baby or even an iron deficiency. Make sure that you are getting all of the vitamins and nutrients that your body needs during pregnancy and that you find a comfortable sleeping position. Be gentle on yourself before bed, finding relaxing and soothing habits.

**104** Forgetfulness is a common side-effect of pregnancy, often referred to as "pregnancy brain". It isn't clear what causes it, but you may feel very absent-minded at the beginning stages and final stages of your pregnancy. Write things down or email yourself lists so that you don't forget important things. Once the baby is born and you settle into a normal routine, you should find yourself back to normal.

## RELATIONSHIPS

**104** Many couples talk about their love life going out of the window during pregnancy and once the baby is born. When you're exhausted, swollen and uncomfortable, physical intimacy may be the last thing on your mind. However, talking to your partner throughout the process and making time for just the two of you is important. Try to find some passion and romance together so that you feel connected to one another.

**105** Your emotional rollercoaster during pregnancy may leave you fearful of being abandoned or something happening to your partner. Finding yourself becoming clingy is normal as you feel more and more responsible for the baby growing inside of you. Talk through your fears with your partner and share your concerns. He probably has some of his own to share with you too.

**106** Finances can put strain on a relationship when a baby is on the way. It's no longer just you two to take care of and that can be a scary and overwhelming thought. Your partner may feel as though it is his duty to provide for the family and may experience stress if he doesn't feel as though he can. Visit a financial advisor as a couple and make it clear to your partner that you are in the situation together.

**107** Relationships with your support network such as your family and friends may strengthen during pregnancy and the birthing process as you enter a different phase in your life. You will be able to relate more to the family and friends who have had children and they, in turn, will offer you the advice and support that you need. Cherish this network.

**108** You may find, however, that relationships with friends who do not have children change. When your single friends are bar-hopping and you're at home changing diapers, it's difficult to find common ground. If you're feeling unsupported by any of your friends, talk to them about what you are experiencing and let them talk to you about how they feel about you having a baby. The good friends will find a way to be there for you.

# CHAPTER 7 – APPROACHING THE BIG DAY

**109** Once you have decided on your healthcare practitioner, you will put together a birth plan where you will decide the environment that you want to give birth in, how you feel about pain medication, muscle relaxants, epidurals and other drugs during birth, the type of hydration you'd prefer during the process, the type of monitoring, labor induction, pushing, delivery and what happens immediately following delivery. Ensure that you are completely comfortable with your birth plan and discuss it thoroughly with your practitioner.

**110** Finances have been discussed before, but before the big day ensure that you have a baby budget that makes provisions for all of the new expenses that you are going to incur including clothes, toys, blankets, food and diapers.

**111** Put together a list of your favorite baby names with your partner so that when you see him or her for the first time, you have a few ideas for names that you agree on.

**112** During pregnancy, it's important to shop for maternity clothes and underwear as your belly grows. These clothes will be comfortable for you after birth as well, as the swelling gradually reduces. You may take a few months to lose the baby weight as well so don't be too hard on yourself when it comes to fitting into your normal clothes too soon.

**113** Throw a baby shower or ask one of your friends or family members to organize one for you. This is not only a fun day out where the focus is on you and your baby, but you'll get some great baby gifts too. There are many fun themes and games that you can play and a baby registry will ensure that you receive all of the items that you need.

**114** If you are planning on breastfeeding after you give birth, learn as much as you can about it as it's not always an easy process. Speak to other mothers, read up about and ask your healthcare practitioner for advice.

**115** Get your home baby-proofed and ready for him or her. Decorate and stock baby's room so that everything is ready for the big day. Lock away medicines and sharp objects, put up baby gates if you have stairs and ensure that the cot or crib is secure.

**116** If you are planning on returning to work soon after giving birth, start doing some research on childcare options. You want to leave your baby with someone that you trust completely so take some time to find the right person.

**117** Take a tour of the hospital or birthing center before the big day so that you know what to expect and where to go when you arrive. This will help you to feel more comfortable when you eventually do get there.

**118** Have a bag packed and ready for the hospital or birthing center. You may go into labor earlier than expected so ensure that you have everything that you need including a toothbrush and toothpaste, comfortable clothes, a hair brush and other home comforts is ready to go. Have your healthcare practitioner's number on speed dial.

**119** Choose a pediatrician who will treat your baby after he or she is born by doing some research and tapping into your support network.

# CHAPTER 8 – THE BIG DAY

**119** As the big day approaches, you will start to feel heavier as the baby moves further down in your uterus. You may experience more severe back aches and be more tired than usual. Your healthcare practitioner will advise you on what to do once you start experiencing contractions but once they become more regular and intense, it is time to head to the hospital or birthing center.

**120** Your waters may break, which is a sign that you are in labor, however it only occurs in less than 20% of births so don't wait for it to happen to be sure. When in doubt, call your healthcare practitioner or go through to the birthing center or hospital anyway. Rather be safer than sorry.

**121** If your baby is showing no signs of popping out anytime soon, your healthcare professional may decide to induce labor. This is simply the artificial start of labor and usually occurs if the baby is overdue and has not arrived by 42 weeks. However, labor may also be induced if your waters have broken too early or there is a health problem with the baby. Usually a pill or a gel is used to induce labor.

**122** You will either have a natural, vaginal birth or a Caesarean section. The ultimate goal is the safety and optimum health of you and the baby.

C-Sections are often planned if a natural birth won't be safe for the baby or if there is more than one baby or if it is preferred by the mother. Emergency C-sections may occur if the baby gets stuck or is not in the right position. Women with small pelvises may also need a C-section. Decide with your healthcare practitioner on what is best for you and the baby.

**123** A natural birth can take a long time as you have to wait for your cervix to fully dilate before you can start pushing. You may experience fear and pain during the process so be sure to have your partner and other loved ones around. Walking around or lying in a hot bath may ease the pain from the contractions. You may opt not to have any medication or to have an epidural, which will numb your stomach. It is completely up to you to decide on this.

**124** If you have a C-Section, you will undergo anesthesia, which will numb your abdomen. You will be awake, but there will be a curtain over your mid-section, so you won't see what is going on. It should be a fairly quick process but due to the surgery, you will take longer to recover.

**125** Once your baby is born, you will get to hold him or her for the first time. It's okay if you feel a little bit groggy. You can choose to have him or her washed after the birth as well as who will cut the cord.

**126** Allow the nurses to help you to feed and wash your baby during the first few days while you recover. Lean on your partner and the support of friends and family too. Try to get lots of rest before you head home.

# CHAPTER 9 – FIRST 6 MONTHS AFTER

## SLEEP

**127** Your newborn baby will want to feed often – every two to three hours, which may take a toll on your sleeping pattern. You also may need to wake your baby up to feed him or her. Set an alarm to help get you up every few hours and try to have regular naps during the day, when the baby is napping, to catch up on sleep.

**128** It will take a little while to get used to your newborn's cries and understand what they mean so it's okay to feel a bit frustrated in the beginning, especially when you're being woken up often. This is perfectly normal.

**129** Over the course of the next few weeks, you'll start settling into a routine but doing what you can to get baby to sleep including rocking him or her or even letting the baby sleep in the bed with you. After a few months, however, you'll need to get baby into a good sleeping pattern in his or her crib. It's important that baby learns to fall asleep in his or her crib without needing you there to do so.

**130** It is recommended that baby sleeps in a crib in your room for the first six months so you can be close to him or her for feeding. Newborns also need a lot of attention and love. After six months, baby should be ready to move into the nursery.

**131** Swaddling your baby is a good way to recreate the snug environment of your womb, helping him or her to sleep soundly. It is recommended to put your baby on his or her back in a secure space so that no rolling will occur.

**132** Your baby might make some strange noises while he or she sleeps, which is perfectly normal. However, if you hear wheezing or grunting or baby seems to be breathing abnormally, call your pediatrician immediately.

## TIME MANAGEMENT

**133** Your body is still undergoing massive changes when you bring your baby home and you may find that you are overwhelmed by the lack of sleep and constant feeding, bathing and changing of baby. Housework, cooking, washing clothes and even showering may take second priority.

**134** Ask friends and family to help you with meals over the first few weeks after your baby is born. They can draw up a roster between them and you can freeze the dinners that you don't finish. This will make it far easier to eat nutritional and wholesome meals when you have little time to cook.

**135** Hire a house cleaner or use a laundry service during the first few months, taking the pressure off you while you learn the ins and outs of parenthood. This will free up time for you to look after yourself and your baby.

**136** Prioritize what is important every single day and let the rest go. In the first few weeks, baby and sleep are going to be top priorities. Work out a routine with your partner so that you each have tasks to focus on.

**137** Break up the tasks over the week so you don't feel overwhelmed each day. On day one, just worry about a clean kitchen. On day two, just worry about a clean living room. It will feel far more manageable.

**138** Be gentle on yourself. You aren't going to have it all figured out on day one. You're going to have to be flexible with your schedule and understand that you are fitting in with baby's routine, not the other way round, for just a little while.

## Social Life

**139** Just because your life has turned upside down doesn't mean that your social life has to come to an abrupt halt. Invite another new mom over for tea and swap stories while the babies nap. It will make you feel less alone and provide you with some much needed friend-time.

**140** Your mother and his mother might be far too eager to help but let them. Allow them to watch the baby for an hour while you join a friend for a jog or go out for dinner with your partner. It's important to connect with other adults during this time.

**141** Join a mommy yoga class to lose your baby weight and get to know other moms. Exercise will increase your endorphins while the group around you will know exactly what you are going through.

**142** You may feel like a bit of an alien compared to your childless friends, but invite them over to meet the baby and get comfortable with the situation – they may be babysitting for you sometime after all. Watch a movie, share some tea and cake and talk to each other about what is going on in each other's lives. This will help you to feel as though you are still close to your friends, even if some things have changed.

**143** You and your partner need to make some time for each other, even if it's a romantic dinner while the baby is napping. Your relationship will still need some love and attention so try to enjoy quality time as a couple too.

## ME TIME

**144** For the first time in your life, you have a little being to care for who is entirely your responsibility. It's a daunting task and you may feel as though you are never doing enough for your newborn. It's important, however, to look after yourself too so that you can give your baby the very best of you.

**145** Take some time to exercise after you given birth so that you lose your baby weight quickly and feel good about how you are looking. Go for a walk with the baby in the stroller, join an exercise class or sign-up to a running club.

**146** It's easy and understandable to want to remain in your pajamas all day but try to get into a routine of showering, doing your hair and getting dressed each day. You will feel fresh and more awake.

**147** Get some rest and sleep as often as you can. Midwives and doctors often suggest sleeping when the baby sleeps and there is a reason for this. Especially if you are recovering from a C-section, you need your sleep.

**148** Talk to your doctor or pediatrician whenever you have any concerns rather than worrying about it. You don't need the added stress of imagining the worst when you already have so much on your plate.

**149** Invest in some good quality headphones and some soothing music. The ability to shut the world out and spend some time in a state of calmness can not only be a rewarding treat but can also help to stop and reflect on the experience, as a whole.

**150** Be firm with people when it comes to your time. They will sometimes forget how important it is to you right now. You don't need to be rude about it but you will need to put the foot down, from time to time. Remember, it's OK to put you first, even if you are not used to doing it.

# CONCLUSION

It is estimated by UNICEF that 353 000 babies are born every single day all over the world. You are not alone.

Your support network of family and friends, your partner and the team of professionals around you are there to make the transition into parenthood as easy as possible. It's not always going to be easy, sometimes you will be afraid and other times you will feel as though you're drowning. Most times, however, you are going to feel overwhelming joy when you experience life with the infant that you and your partner have created.

Nine months is a long time to be pregnant but it is the preparation time that you need before baby becomes a part of your life. Look after yourself, nurture your relationship with your partner, nourish your body with good and wholesome foods, get enough rest and most importantly, enjoy it.

With these tips, hacks and advice, you should be set to go. Good luck on this beautiful and exciting journey.

# DID YOU ENJOY THIS BOOK?

I want to thank you for purchasing and reading this book. I really hope you got a lot out of it.

Can I ask a quick favor though?

If you enjoyed this book I would really appreciate it if you could leave me a positive review on Amazon.

I love getting feedback from my customers and reviews on Amazon really do make a difference. I read all my reviews and would really appreciate your thoughts.

Thanks so much.

Taryn Accardo

# ABOUT THE AUTHOR

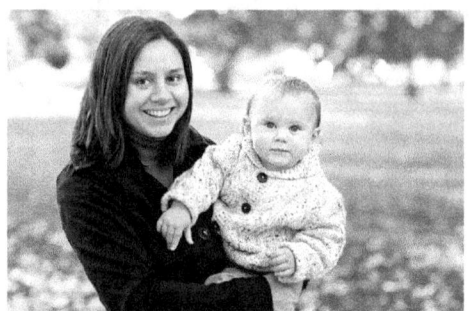

**Taryn Accardo** is a wife, mother, researcher and author, who loves to write about the things that fascinate her. She has a passion for sharing here knowledge and experience and genuinely enjoys helping others through education and encouragement. Taryn brings real-world experience into her writings, not only from her own journey but from that of others. She believes it is important to impart knowledge but it's far better to impart wisdom.